The Light of Chi

Denise Richard

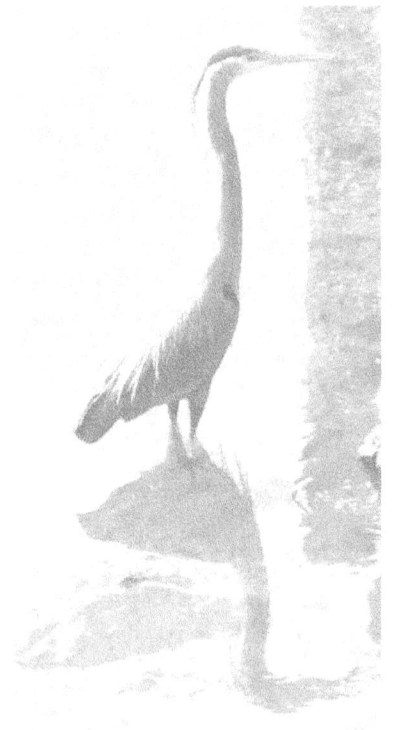

ISBN – 13:978-1537491059
ISBN-10: 1537491059

DEDICATION

This little book is dedicated to the graceful teacher that guided me to know the Light of Chi. To my Sifu Juiling Peng for all his love and understanding.

CONTENTS

ACKNOWLEDGMENTS

I say thank you to those who have held the Light of Chi in the most arduous of practices. The way of Chi Kung is held in my heart as it serves to open to compassion and service. To all my teachers I acknowledge the immense beauty of your presence. To the Grand Masters who have held my heart I love you always.

1. THE LIGHT OF CHI AND THE FIELD OF CONSCIOUSNESS

In this work we look to Chi Kung as a distinct way of healing. The practice of Chi Kung enables the opening of channels that hold the Light of Chi. As channels are free of challenge, the movement of Chi engages the exchange of energy and the holding of health. This way is effortless and naturally protects the body as the flow is supported through the field.

The process of healing is not the traditional movement of presence. What Chi Kung offers is a simple exchange with the light of consciousness to support the letting go of pain. In this way the focus is to hold awareness of light and allow the healing of distress. With this effortless way we do not look to manipulate or control. The view is simply that the light field is the wise counsel that knows the greater good and looks to support the heart.

The way of Chi Kung offers a sensitive view of consciousness that understands that the management of energy is based in the light body. At the highest level we see that consciousness is the knowing of a huge power that guides this world. Those who look to the natural world as a place of refuge know that the light of consciousness is healthy in those who secure and protect nature. The respect we share for that which nurtures and protects us is our home.

When looking for support we know that there is a distant need for security. Those who look for this practice are held to work with their physical and subtle bodies to help maintain a generous attitude of service and connection. The exchange is visible as the practitioner needs to serve community and helps to protect the field that holds the healthy light. The practice of Chi Kung helps to awaken the body and supports the flow of healing light at all levels.

What we recognise as we grow in this way is the continuous awakening of the bodymind. The practice is deep intelligence of an ancient making. The growth of the field is at once a personal and micro consciousness that allows for service and healing. This field is recognised as purity and holds no bounds.

2. THE LIGHT OF CHI

The tradition of Chinese health management discovered long ago that in cultivating Chi there was a special process through which energy was transmuted into consciousness. The term for this process of transmutation is called alchemy. Taoist masters realized this understanding through centuries of study and observation of the energy flow in the plexus areas of the body. Energy in the plexus of the pelvis, heart and head is stabilized and held as a resource to support change.

With this understanding the student who learns the ancient art of Chi Kung is taught to develop energy and transform it into consciousness; for as Chi builds in the body the next step is for the alchemy of the heart to take place. Chi rises into the heart plexus and then becomes the agent through which the heart is refined, opened and clarified. As this happens a clear light appears in the heart plexus and it becomes the foundation for awareness. Taoist practice therefore supports the clearing and opening of heart and the awakening of consciousness through the building of a strong and stable energy system.

The body is the vehicle through which consciousness is developed. By practicing simple and precise movements, the energy system becomes infused with Chi and begins to relax. Just like a child who is held in the arms of a loving mother, the practitioner of Taoist arts learns that a greater force is present and available to help hold, nourish and heal within the surrounding environment.

There is a shift in consciousness that gently and slowly occurs as the student can open to greater harmony with community and heart. When these work together deep changes can take place for all systems are interconnected. Taoist practice brings not only the gift of harmony, security and health, but it also provides the link of awareness.

For the new student it will take time and consistent application in order for new patterns of flow and health to take root. The most significant change will present itself as new depth of quietness and keener observation. As a practitioner of over 25 years I can attest to the beauty, the grace and healing consciousness of Chi Kung.

The light of Chi presents itself through the realization of ones' true nature; this is a quality of beauty that is reflected through heartfelt presence. When this level of presence is attained there is an experience of a deep love for the earth and all that is natural. As the light of heart is awakened the pure consciousness of the natural world draws us, feeds us and supports harmonious relationship. When people gather to practice Taoist arts there is a synergy that occurs where the Light of Chi collectively pools to offers a container in which the student can grow. The gentleness and simplicity of the practices allow for deep relaxation and depth of awareness revealing the internal wisdom and brilliance of the body. For those looking towards the natural world with reverence and a passion for awakening consciousness, the Taoist path speaks profound truth.

3. DEVOTIONAL PRACTICE

Thousands of years of spiritual life have brought us to know that the service of our hearts leads to the actual placement in the light of consciousness.

In many traditions we learn that the offering of will to that which is greater and of total understanding brings a knowing of that. In experience we come to see this as the ultimate gift to giving. Giving of heart, will and mind is sometimes called surrender. This is the common thread we find in all spiritual people.

When we encounter a process where pain and suffering engage our sensitivity to the conflicts we have between the working physical world and the loving spiritual world we are sitting at the edge of our spiritual understanding. The ability to know how to let go and allow the greater light to secure and protect is of the upmost value. The teaching is active as the process of our consciousness is of choice. To devote and hold reverence and respect for that which is good will be the one way to know.

Devotion is the active process of total surrender that places us in a mutual experience of respect. Therefore in this place the boundaries that unify and ask us to know the play of spirituality are sensitively guided through the one who has been designated. Those who look to the teacher as the one who has dominion will lose the understanding of the devotional field of goodness.

Therefore when we hold devotion of a high nature we come to know others of a loving way also sensitive of heart. We come to recognise that the world we know is good when those that surround us can claim a personal field that is of great health and bountifully held in acceptance.

4. THE STUDENT

When the student has decided and knows that the path is chosen the process of transformation takes on a will of its own. Nothing can prepare us for the amount of power and process that will come since it is guided by something well beyond our physical nature. The Light of Chi is not something that we can control it's a divine resource that moves through our own consciousness by way of allowing it. The practice is of knowing that this permission is something that we might need to work with since this culture is so dedicated to dominance and control. To witness someone simply follow and allow the momentum of a process to unfold without resistance can seem ludicrous to some. The path of least resistance is known in Taoism to be the one path that can support the light without effort.

There is a lot that I can say about how the path is strong for those who commit. It's not a given that all will achieve the Light of Chi. It is a given that all will understand the strength and open heart required when moved to act without consciousness. For this is the main issue that everyone faces on a spiritual path. The light is not a doctor, it's a momentum that works us to understand and hold our own value system. For this reason the teacher is the most important person on the path because they support the managing of the chi and the difficulties at the most sensitive junctions. The light of Chi is not an easy power to move with when the consciousness is not of heart. What a person requires is the knowledge of self in a greater way; the light will always be available to those who seek.

MASTER AND LIGHT

To those who know the way there is mastery. As the practice becomes us, we become a field of understanding. The honour of knowing the light of consciousness and having the respect of those who hold our hand is given. What the guide offers is clarity of reflection in life process; for together the work helps to secure those who look to know, as there is continuous learning.

FIVE BLOSSOMS

Five blossoms of
Light pink scent
With fields placing
Thought in sunshine

Gathering softly on
Ponds of clear
Light reflecting that
Wonder and joy

The gem found
Roaring with awareness
Since life exhilarates
In dew drop

ABOUT THE AUTHOR

With three decades of practice & support in the field of Chi Kung and energy management Denise Richard is a qualified instructor of an ancient system of health and healing. Her long standing experience has brought her to know this delicate understanding of the Light of Chi that holds great service to you.

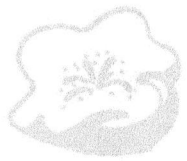

www.fiveblossomgatherings.com